# Broken Trust
# When Cries for Help Are Not Heard

## Mary Karol, Author

**2020 © Survive a Stroke Foundation**

**All rights reserved**

# Dedication Page

To Rose, my Mom, who should have been a survivor of a medical emergency. Her memory has been the inspiration for this booklet. No one in her skilled nursing facility called 911. No one in the hospital provided medical care. This booklet is for Rose. To help readers as they age learn how to prepare for any kind of medical emergency.

*Sophocles. Electra:  Foolish is the child who forgets a parent's piteous death.*

# About the Author

The author, Mary Karol, is a former graduate law school professor, a frequent speaker for continuing education, and published in numerous business journals. She is active in estate planning and elder law organizations. She wrote this booklet to be an informative and easy read for anyone, but particularly for those who are growing older or have aging family members. Donations from this booklet go to the Survive a Stroke Foundation.

The author **updated the booklet in 2020** to provide information for readers to learn how to prepare and protect themselves and those they love as they age post COVID-19 pandemic. Growing older is now a challenge in the U.S.

# Strokes are Sneaky
# You Don't Know When
# They Will Appear

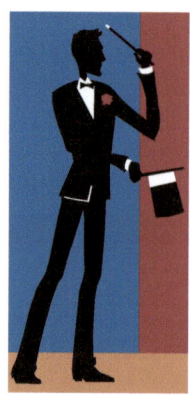

# Table of Contents

Introduction   Pg 6

Part One:  Pictures Tell the Story of a Stroke   Pg 8

Part Two:  The Story of Rose   Pg 23

Part Three: Advance Directives and POLST   Pg 27

Part Four:  Remember What Happened to Rose Pg 37

Disclaimer: Page 45

# Introduction

This easy to read and understand illustrated booklet will help you, or someone you love, survive a stroke and other medical emergencies. Why is this critical to learn today? Medical emergencies can happen at any time. You don't get a second chance very often to recognize and respond to a stroke. It is an example of a medical emergency that is common as people age, and may now even occur with younger persons.

In 2020 it was discovered that even though typically considered a lung infection, COVID-19 has been found to cause blood clots that can lead to severe stroke.  Experts say that this can happen in any patient regardless of age, and even in those with few or no symptoms.

Think of someone you just spoke with or spent time with today. No warning.  They cannot tell you they need help. They cannot tell anyone that something is wrong.  Their cries for help will not be heard. They may even have medical personnel around them who do nothing.  Precious time starts slipping by.

This booklet is based on a true story. It can happen to anyone unable to help themselves in a medical emergency. You cannot count on the health care system to help you. Read on and you will understand why the trust in that system is broken.

Everyone should recognize the signs of a stroke. Any of the stroke symptoms in Part One is a reason to call 911. Don't rely on others to diagnose what is and is not a stroke in progress. Many residential or care facilities for seniors may not respond. **Medical neglect is common**. Do not rely on them.

People have been turned away from emergency rooms when they arrive as a nonemergency call with family or friends. A potential stroke is an emergency. **Be warned** - the older a person is, the less attention they may receive in the ER for any condition. Even age 65 may be considered to be "old". Younger persons in the ER will get more attention.

This booklet provides critical information about advance directives, a POLST, and a needed questionnaire and checklist for medical care as a person ages. Life or death decisions may have to be made for someone you love, or someone has to make for you.

If you are growing older – and that can mean even as young as age 65 - or you have an underlying medical condition - do not trust the health care system to look out for your best interests. There are still a few good people working as health care providers – but hard to find. The US is going corporate and uncaring toward those who are aging or in frail health.

# Part One

# Pictures Tell the Story of a Stroke : Lessons to be Learned Now, While There is Time

What are the warning signs that a stroke has started?

Look over the illustrations below and remember them. If any of these happen, you should be put on notice and ready to call 911 immediately!!

Look at each of the following examples and do not ignore any of them if they happen. Any one of these can be the signal of a stroke. Many think that a stroke has to have a droopy face. That is not true. Do not wait for someone else to make the decision that something is wrong. No matter where you are, others may make a mistake and do nothing. Do not hesitate to act and do not be embarrassed. You are recognizing an emergency!
If you don't act, the consequences are often death or disability for you or the ones you love.

# #1
## Sudden Event  or Change ?

You, or someone you are with, all of a sudden undergoes a sudden unexplained change ?
This can be a stroke !

# #2
# Confused ?

You, or someone you are with, all of a sudden becomes confused ? This can be a stroke !

# #3
# Headache ?

You, or someone you are with, all of a sudden has a terrible headache ? This can be a stroke !

# #4
# Trouble Speaking or Not Speaking ?

You, or someone you are with, all of a sudden has trouble talking or isn't talking at all ? This can be a stroke !

# #5
# Cannot Swallow Easily ?

You, or someone you are with, all of a sudden has trouble swallowing their pills, drink or food ?  This can be a stroke !

# #6
# Paralyzed or Droopy ?

You, or someone you are with, all of a sudden has an arm, leg or side of the face become droopy or paralyzed ?  This can be a stroke !

# Any of those six examples can signal a stroke and the clock starts ticking

## Time to Act Fast – Every Minute Counts

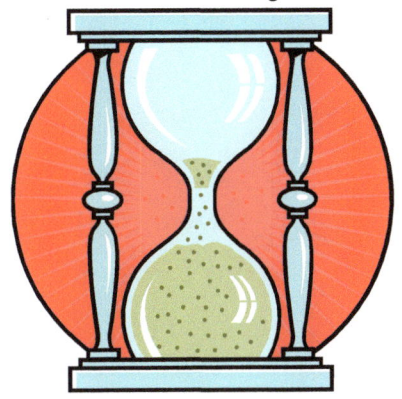

## Telephone Right Away

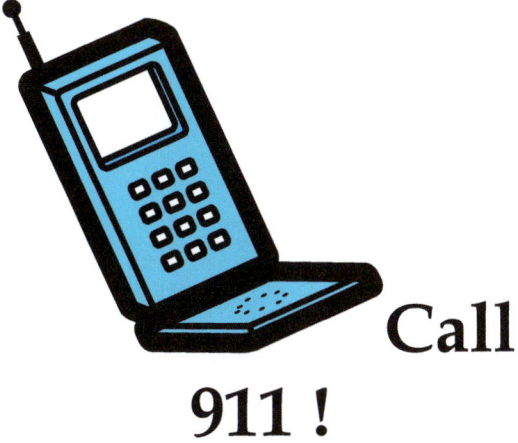

# Call 911 !

# Get An Ambulance to the Nearest Hospital

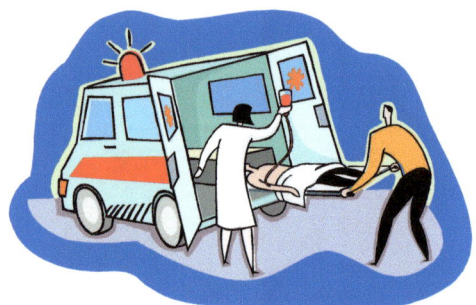

Get to a hospital emergency room (ER) in an ambulance. Do not drive to the ER.

A stroke is an emergency and will be given the highest priority by the emergency room at the hospital when an ambulance brings you. The emergency response team in an ambulance will call in to the ER that they may have a stroke victim, so the ER is prepared to act when you arrive.

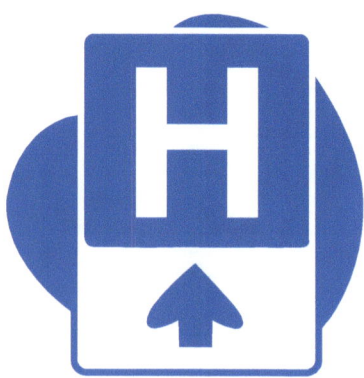

In the Emergency Room the doctors can determine if it's a stroke and if there is a blood clot or if it's bleeding in the brain.

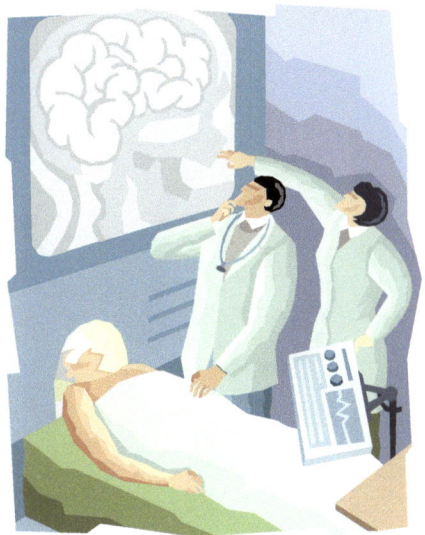

A drug can be injected within 3-4 hours after a stroke if there is a clot to break up the clot. The brain starts to die every minute that it is deprived of blood flow for oxygen. And, if you cannot make that 3-4 hour window, there still is time.

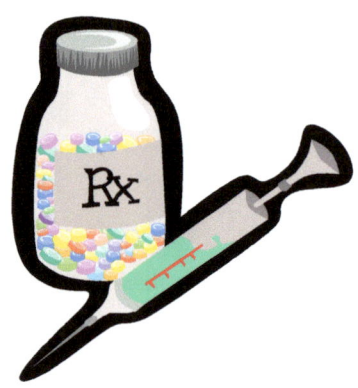

Don't let that precious window of time pass. Up to 8 hours after the onset of a stroke, there are still procedures that can save a life !

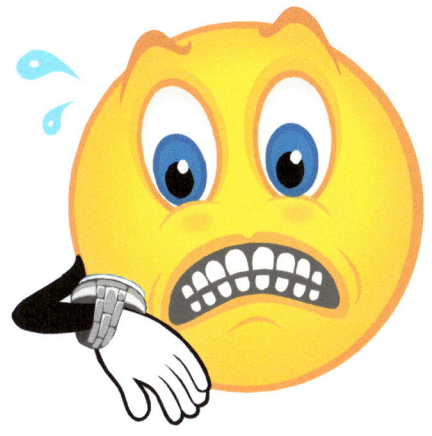

If needed, the hospital ER will have you airlifted to a hospital that is certified as an acute primary stroke center after you are stabalized.  Primary stroke centers are prepared to treat acute stroke victims.

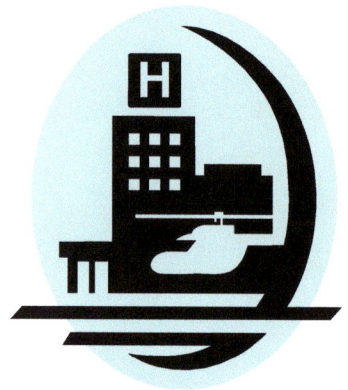

Don't end up with a broken heart because no one called 911 in time. Don't rely on the decisions or actions of others – they can be wrong.

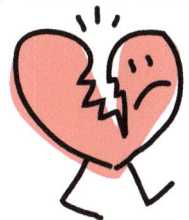

Don't say good bye to the ones you love because no one called 911.

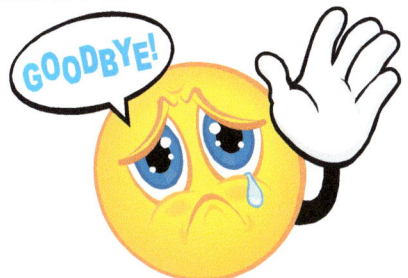

There is no reason for a person to die from a stroke who could have been saved.  If it is someone you love, its very painful.
**Stroke is one of the leading causes of death in the United States. It has been linked in 2020 to COVID-19  for persons of all ages.**

A stroke not recognized and treated properly, if it doesn't cause a death, may cause a serious disability. **Stroke is a leading cause of disability in the United States. It can put you in a nursing home for years.**

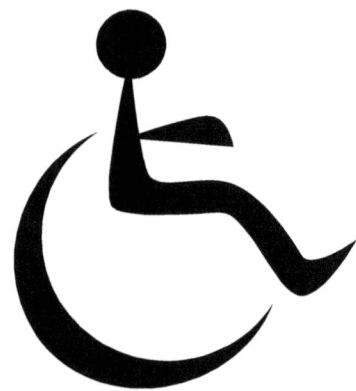

Don't Let this Happen To You or To Someone You Love.

# Part Two

# The Story of Rose

Help Me! .. Help Me!!
Motionless unable to move in her bed, Rose pleaded for
help. Didn't anyone hear her?
Rose could see the people – why didn't they see she needed
help?
Daytime, nighttime, they just looked right past her.
Didn't anyone care? Was no one going to help her?
Rose's family found her there abandoned and knew she
needed help. They called for an ambulance to take her to
the emergency room at a hospital. It was only two minutes
away. Why hadn't the nursing home staff sent her to the
ER?
Rose waited in the emergency room with her family, trying
to tell anyone what had happened to her. Rose was so
relieved to be at the hospital where someone surely would
help her. She smiled at the doctor and the nurses.

But the doctor was not smiling. Rose had come from a
skilled nursing facility, a "nursing home". The doctor
shook his head and sighed. "Oh yes" he said, this is what is
happening now. The nursing homes don't always recognize
a medical emergency. They ignore the cries for help. They
don't call for an ambulance when it's needed. They don't
send older residents to the hospital. They don't care.
The doctor was cold when he spoke to Rose and her family.
It was shocking that way he treated Rose.

The doctor suspected Rose had suffered a stroke but he said nothing. He admitted her to a low level general care floor in the hospital with no special instructions for care.

For 19 days Rose fought to stay alive against the worst odds. The option for care and recovery in the hospital were not offered even **when she asked for help**. Rose left this world early one morning and is sorely missed by those who love her.

## WHAT SHOULD HAVE HAPPENED BESIDES THE NURSING HOME CALLING 911?

Frightening isn't it? These are the health care providers who are licensed by the state to provide care for their residents and patients. Baby boomers fear ending their life in a nursing home, and for good reason. There are good nursing homes, but often not the ones that the majority of seniors can afford. And stay at home services for seniors? They must make sure their clients have their medical care instructions in an obvious place where they can be found quickly; and they must train their staff to recognize medical emergencies and know what to call 911!

This is the true story of Rose, a senior, who died after 19 days from complications from a survivable stroke. Why?

#1 The health care providers in a "skilled" nursing home did not call 911. They did not send her to the ER. They followed a state order not to send older residents to the ER.

#2 The POLST form in Rose's file was over 4 years old and filled out in a rush by the "skilled" nursing home.

Her **old POLST** form was not reviewed by the health care providers (not even the hospital) with Rose or her family when her **condition changed**. It no longer reflected the type of care that Rose wanted.  They were not interested in helping her live. With proper care, Rose would have had a chance to survive. If there had been any discussion by the health care providers with the family about the old POLST and Rose's current condition, all choices to keep Rose alive would have been made.
**Don't let strangers make these life or death decisions for someone you love.**

Health care personnel are supposed to do everything possible to keep a patient alive in the event of a medical emergency. **Unfortunately, they do not always do that with older patients.**  Once a person reaches the age of 65 years, or has any underlying health issues, they may be classified as vulnerable and in the "at risk" group. **This can mean they are denied the care they should receive and want to receive.**

The  **Centers for Disease Control and Prevention (CDC)** states that vulnerable populations may include anyone who has difficulty communicating, has difficulty accessing medical care, may need help maintaining independence, requires constant supervision, or may need help accessing transportation.

Everyone as they grow older, or those who have underlying health issues, the "at risk" group, should have an advance directive, and a POLST if in the later stages of their life.

In addition, there should be clear written **current** instructions on a checklist or other written document in which the person is clear on what they want for their medical care. Discussion on a regular basis with those persons who will have to help that older or vulnerable person when there is a medical emergency. Remember, older may mean even age 65 !

A current complete HIPPA form for medical access should be in place at all times for the person and for those authorized on the form to have immediate access to the information. When a medical crisis happens, loved ones may be shut out and unable to help if the needed forms are not already in place and current. If there is a conflict between the documents, the most recent one takes precedence. Confusion and disagreements on medical care between health care providers and family should not occur if documents are clear and current.

**Find out what ongoing care is needed after a medical emergency in order for a person to survive, rather than having a slow decline to death. Demand the details that will help your loved one live. Know your rights. The health care providers will not volunteer this information for older or vulnerable patients.**

# Part Three

## Advance Directives and POLST

At any age, a medical emergency can leave a person too ill to make his or her own health care decisions. Typically health care choices are documented in living wills and/or durable powers of attorney for health care. **These are referred to as advance directives and are not intended to be end of life instructions.** Often they are done as a part of an estate plan.  As a person ages, or has a serious health condition, they may be forced to sign a POLST. This is a medical order and is critical as an added planning tool to be used with any advance directives to clarify the type of care wanted in a medical emergency or a possible end of life condition. But even with these documents, there can be serious problems receiving the proper care for an older or vulnerable person, the "at risk" group, with a medical emergency.

In the United States alone, more than half a million reports of medical neglect, professional negligence and elder abuse reach authorities every year, and many incidents go unreported.  Most are settled out of court and the public never hears the true story. Frequently the claims are for the health care provider's failure to follow advance directives and/or a POLST. **A person in the "at risk" group may have their wishes for medical care ignored. Elder abuse includes being denied medical care.**

It is important to realize that this can happen. You must learn now how to prevent these life or death failures from happening. If you are a health care agent for someone you love, you must know what to do to be a strong advocate. You must defend and protect your loved one's rights for medical care if they want to survive. Do not count on the system to help you as you age. You are considered more of a liability then an asset as you grow older.

## Advance Directives

Advance directives are legal documents.

The living will, also known as a physician's directive, is one type of advance directive. This documents a person's desires for treatment in the event of a medical emergency. The living will is typically signed when a person is younger, healthy, and able to make his/her own decisions. However, the decisions made years before on a living will "form" may not reflect the person's true thoughts about their medical care in later years. Living wills are available online as a form and may not be completed correctly by a lay person.

A durable power of attorney for health care is another type of advance directive. It is a type of durable power of attorney which allows a person to name someone else as his/her health care agent (surrogate) to oversee his/her medical care and to make health care decisions for them if they are unable to do so at any time.

These too are available online as a form and may not be completed correctly by a person. They are best completed in a lawyer's office.

## POLSTs

The POLST started in Oregon in 1991, when those concerned with medical ethics discovered that patient preferences for their end of life care were not consistently followed.

See the contact information: National Polst Task Force website **http://www.polst.org/about-the-national-polst-paradigm.**

The POLST is a medical order, not a legal document. Because it was created only in the 1990's, there are fewer statutes and reported cases on POLST than advance directives. POLST forms are appropriate for individuals with a serious illness or advanced frailty near the end of life. The POLST is intended to add to, not replace, an advance directive for those persons near the end of life.

The POLST form is to be kept at the front of a health care patient or resident's file, or in a visible place such as the refrigerator door at home if the person is still residing at home. In a medical emergency it is available to first responders and travels with the patient.

The use of POLST forms can overcome many of the problems associated with advance directives.

Advance directives in many cases are completed simply to name an individual to make health care decisions for the patient if the latter becomes incapacitated and the advance directive "form" may lack specificity in regard to the patient's health care preferences.

Advance directives are often locked away in file drawers or safe deposit boxes and unavailable to health care providers when the need arises to ensure that the patient's wishes are followed.

Lay persons are generally not familiar with the POLST and do not understand that the decisions on this form are for life or death in a medical emergency or change in condition. If signing for a person as their health care agent under a durable power of attorney for health care, a complete understanding of the form is needed before signing. This should be a time for serious and thoughtful discussion.

Unfortunately for medical care or end of life planning, the POLST too may have its failures. For instance, the POLST should not be signed too early.

Often the POLST is **signed in a rush** in a nursing home, by a hospice team member, the visiting nurse, or for those with home health care services. There is little or no discussion. How can anyone make life or death decisions in a rush?

As an example and warning, the **Attorney General's office of Louisiana** gave a formal opinion on some of the problems that can arise with a POLST. This is a rare example of a good protective provision in State law. Specifically mentioned was a nursing home or a hospital where elderly and/or other patients are admitted and routinely approached by physicians or other health care providers who seek to write up a POLST on them for the future, and ask that the person to make an "end-of-life" declaration in order to complete the POLST.

This is a violation of state law in **Louisiana** which provides: "A person shall not be required to make a declaration as a condition for being insured or *for receiving health care services, and* in order to avoid such a violation of law, the patient should first be made to understand that he or she does not have to make any "end-of-life" declaration. *The person may be ninety years old but suffers from nothing but elderly age."*

Another problem addressed with the POLST is that there are **no formal execution requirements**. Who can witness, notarize or verify the person understood what they signed? Life or death medical care decisions must be understood and explained before signing a POLST.

A POLST is signed by the patient (or person with a durable power of attorney for health care) and in most states that provide for a POLST, a health care professional (usually a physician, advance nurse practitioner, or physician assistant) must also sign.

The definition of who is a health care professional for purposes of the POLST form varies from state to state; but in all states that have adopted the POLST it is an immediate actionable medical order when completed.

**Not all health care professionals are trained in explaining end of life decisions that are made on a POLST, and many do not care about the "at risk group" patient at all.**

In one case, a nurse departed from the applicable standard of care when she failed to respond within an hour or two to the initial fax sent regarding the patient's symptoms and then consult with a physician. The nurse's unsuccessful defense in part was that the patient's POLST requested only comfort care. The patient died.

In another case, a California physician had a high volume geriatric practice with many patients from long-term care facilities. The physician claimed he could not be liable under the Elder Abuse Act for failure to follow or update the POLST because he was not the patient's custodian or caretaker. The patient died.

**One of the biggest failures with a POLST is when it is not kept current.**

This is a very large problem in nursing homes with untrained and low skilled staff,  and also may occur with stay at home senior services.

The POLST can become outdated and produce the wrong life or death result.  If a POLST is not kept current or followed correctly, a person's wishes may evaporate in a medical emergency.

The POLST is to be reviewed, discussed and updated <u>each time</u> there is a change in condition with the patient;

or <u>each time</u> when the patient transfers in and out of  a health care setting (such as from the nursing home to the hospital and back to the nursing home). A POLST remains operative until it is changed or revoked.

Thus, many months or even years may pass after a POLST is on file, during which time the patient's medical condition may change and their desires for medical care will change. **Life becomes more precious with age.**

To emphasize the critical message on survival, if a person has suffered a stroke, or other medical emergency, and cannot speak, how can they tell their health care providers what choices they want for medical care? Their POLST needs to be updated right then. What if they want to live and want help?  **If they are growing older, or in the "at risk" group, they may be denied any medical care.**

The POLST must be updated after discussion with the person's health care agent under their durable power of attorney.

The Federal Nursing Home Reform Act or OBRA '87 created a set of national minimum set of standards of care and rights for people living in certified nursing facilities. Are these really ever followed?

This landmark federal legislation is known as "OBRA" through the legislative process. https://www.govtrack.us/congress/bills/100/hr3545/text.

These quarterly assessments often are done as a mere paperwork meeting to be able to sign off that the assessment was done. No real concern for the resident or follow through in most situations. Don't be fooled. Just try to register a suggestion or complaint with the administrator during these meetings and see how it is ignored! If the patient cannot discuss and make these update decisions, then the person under their durable power of attorney for health care is the party the health care provider must have this discussion with.

OBRA requires nursing homes to conduct assessments for all residents, even if they are not using Medicare or Medicaid to pay for care.

The assessment must be completed when the resident initially enters the nursing home and again every quarter and when the resident is discharged. **In addition, an assessment must be completed if the resident shows a significant change in status or if a correction is made to a previous assessment.**

The quarterly assessment required by a nursing home could also be a good time to review and update a resident's POLST. These are missed opportunities to help elderly residents. The nursing home doesn't care.

If someone does not speak and stand up for the older, or "at risk", person to help them, no one in the health care system will care and do it.  The older your loved one is – or if they fall into the "at risk" group - the less chance they have to receive medical care and help unless you know how to help them. It is a very sad truth for people aging in the United States.

**To stress again the lesson to be learned:**
All persons, as they age, should have current instructions completed for medical care and aging wishes to give to their family, to any person designated as their health care agent under a durable power of attorney, and to their health care provider. A checklist is helpful which can be discussed and which expresses the person's health care, aging, and any end of life wishes to enhance and clarify any advance directives or a POLST.

**Discuss these important life and death decisions.**
Learn through this booklet to be an advocate for yourself
and others.

A checklist can clarify, explain and be kept current so health
care providers can be assured that the choices in the
advance directive and/or POLST are what the person truly
wants.

The checklist can be made a legal part of the advance
directive. A valuable easy to complete questionnaire and
checklist which covers these essential decisions can be
found in the book **Aging in America, a Cautionary Tale of
Wrongful Death in Elder Care. This book is a valuable
resource as you age.**

The **questionnaire and checklist** can be completed in the
book or printed out, and can help begin the important
discussions with friends, family and health care providers.
A current checklist clarifies for others what a person's
wishes are as they age. Go to seniorcare publishing on the
web and enter the code 2019Rose.

Medicare will pay physicians to counsel patients on
advance care and end of life planning. There is a very basic
form many physicians use for this – and have a nurse
practitioner generally meet with the patient.
This is not as thorough a form or appointment as it should
be in most cases.

You must make the effort yourself to make this a meaningful appointment. Don't count on the physician or nurse practitioner.

Medicare covers advance care planning as a separate service provided by physicians and other health care professionals (such as nurse practitioners who bill Medicare using the physician fee schedule). Medicare also covers advance care planning provided in medical offices and facility settings, including hospitals. Advance care and end of life planning encompasses both advance directives and the POLST.

This discussion with the health care professional about an advance directive or POLST is also a good time to go over any completed checklist you have with them. Make sure they know you have a checklist that you keep current.

# Part Four

# Remember What Happened to Rose
# The "At Risk", Vulnerable, Group

**The COVID-19 pandemic of 2019 implemented harmful guidelines for medical care and survival for older persons.**

Influential organizations and individuals produced hospital-care-rationing guidelines that recommend younger people receive higher priority than the elderly during the pandemic, by giving significant weight to how many years of life patients would have ahead of them if treatment is successful. Also, some guidelines bar care-home residents from being transferred to a hospital.

For example, on March 21 the UK's National Institute for Clinical Excellence produced its guidelines. They're based on a frailty score and on mortality probabilities across different age groups for pneumonia and underlying cardiovascular or respiratory diseases.

On March 23 the paper *"Fair allocation of scarce medical resources in the time of Covid-19"* was published in the prestigious NEW ENGLAND JOURNAL OF MEDICINE. The paper's first recommendation calls for:

maximizing the number of patients that survive treatment with a reasonable life expectancy."

On March 27, the equally influential JOURNAL OF THE AMERICAN MEDICAL ASSOCIATION (JAMA) published "A FRAMEWORK FOR RATIONING VENTILATORS AND CRITICAL-CARE BEDS DURING THE COVID-19 PANDEMIC."

The paper's authors assert that:

[y]ounger individuals should receive priority, not because of any claims about social worth or utility, but because they are the worst off, in the sense that they have had the least opportunity to live through life's stages."

Ontario Health published guidelines for hospital-treatment rationing on March 28, albeit not publicly. (To this day the government hasn't made the protocol public, nor disclosed whether or when they implemented it.)

TORONTO STAR reporter Jennifer Yan obtained a copy of the Ontario treatment-triaging document and wrote in a March 29 article that:

[u]nder the triage protocol, long-term-care patients who meet specific criteria will also no longer be transferred to hospitals."

Then on April 10, the Canadian Medical Association adopted all the recommendations by Dr. Ezekiel and his co-authors in their *New England Journal of Medicine* paper, and advised Canadian physicians to follow them.

**Were conditions for high death rates at Care Homes created on purpose? May 26, 2020 -- Sott.net**, researched and reported by Rosemary Frei has an Msc in molecular biology from a faculty of medicine and was a freelance medical writer and journalist for 22 years. She is now an independent investigative journalist.

**Buried in N.Y. Budget: Legal Shield for Nursing Homes Rife With Virus. May 13, 2020 - nytimes.com**. Amy Julia Harris, Kim Barker, Jesse McKinley

In New York, 5,300 nursing home residents have died of Covid-19. The nursing home lobby pressed for a provision that makes it hard for their families to sue.. In the chaotic days of late March, as it became clear that New York was facing a catastrophic outbreak of the coronavirus.

**'They just dumped him like trash': Nursing homes evict vulnerable residents June 21. 2020 - bostonglobe.com**. Jessica Silver-Greenberg, Amy Julia Harris

According to three Lakeview employees, Kendrick's ouster came as the nursing home was telling staff members to try to clear out less-profitable residents to make room for a new class of customers who would generate more revenue: patients with COVID-19. More than any other institution in America, nursing homes have come to symbolize the deadly destruction of the coronavirus crisis.

## HOW TO PREPARE AND PROTECT YOURSELF NOW

**Find out and stay current with the laws in your state and if they will protect you in a medical emergency.**

Be vigilant on **DNR orders** that may have been selected by an older family member on a form.
Do Not Resuscitate (**DNR**), also known as no **code** or allow natural death, choice marked on a form indicates that a person does not want to receive cardiopulmonary resuscitation (CPR) if that person's heart stops beating. Sometimes it also prevents other medical interventions. This can be problem as a person ages and wants medical care in an emergency.

**Health care providers may overlook other choices for medical care when DNR has been chosen. They may presume because a person is "old" that they would want to die.** Health care providers may be younger than an aging patient, and that patient may be viewed as "old" to them.

**A nice "frail" elderly lady the doctors wrote in Rose's file at the hospital. They didn't try to save her. Rose wanted to live and <u>asked for help at the hospital</u>. This is really happening in the United States. Be warned if you are in the "at risk" group now.**

**Health care providers may not follow an advance directives or a POLST.** If your state has these rules, and you are a person's health care agent under a durable power of attorney, you must be prepared ahead of time to demand and fight for your loved one so they receive the medical care they want. In a medical emergency, a person is unlikely to be able to respond to health care providers and fight for their own medical rights.

Texas allows a physician to withhold or withdraw medical treatment requested under a POLST or advance directive if the physician believes it would be futile.
Texas Health and Safety Code, sec 166.046, Texas Advance Directives Act, 1999

In other states, if a health care provider refuses to follow an advance directive or POLST requesting life sustaining measures, the patient must be transferred to a health care provider who will follow the instructions:

Arkansas, Ark. Code Ann. §§ 20-17-207, 20-17-210(f) (2017): Connecticut, Conn. Gen. Stat. §§ 19a-571; 19a580a (West 2016); Guam, 10 Guam Code § 91109 (2016); Illinois,755 Ill. Comp. Stat. Ann. 35/3(d) (West 2016); Iowa, Iowa Code §144A.8 (2016); Kentucky, Ky. Rev. Stat. Ann. §311.633(2) (2017);

Louisiana, La. R.S. §40:1151.6(B), (D) (West 2017); Montana, Mont. Code Ann. §50-9-203 (2017); Nebraska, Neb. Rev. Stat.§ 30-3428(1), (2) (Michie 2016); Nevada, Nev. Rev. Stat. § 449.628 (Michie 2016); New Jersey, N.J. Stat. Ann § 26:2H-65(a)(4)(West 2017); North Carolina, N.C. Gen. Stat. § 90-321(k) (2017) ; North Dakota, N.D. Cent. Code § 23-06.5-12(3) (2016); Oregon, Or. Rev. Stat. § 127.625(2)(c) (2017); Pennsylvania, Pa. Stat. Ann. tit. 20§ 5424 (2016); South Carolina, S.C. Code Ann. § 44-77-100 (2016); Tennessee, Tenn. Code Ann. § 32-11-108 (a) (2016);

Virgin Islands, 19 V.I.C § 193 (2016); Washington, Wash. Rev. Code Ann. §70.122.060(2) (West 2016); West Virginia, W. Va. Code § 16-30-12(a) (2016); and Wisconsin, Wis. Stat. Ann. § 154.07(1)(a) (West 2017)

Ten states require life preserving measures pending a transfer:
Alabama, Ala. Code § 22-8A-8(a)(2017). But: also see Ala. Code § 22-8A-9(d)(2017):Florida, Fla. Stat. Ann. § 765.1105 (1) (2017); Kansas, Kan. Stat. Ann. § 65-28,107(a) (2017); Maryland, Md. Code Ann., [Health-General] § 5-613 (a)(2017); Massachusetts, Mass. Ann. Laws ch. 201D § 14, 15 (Law. Co-op. 2016);

---

Minnesota, Minn. Stat. §145C.15 (2016); New Hampshire, N.H. Rev. Stat. Ann. §137-J:7 (II)(2016); New York, N.Y. [Public Health] Law § 2984(3) (Consol. 2016); Ohio, Ohio Rev. Code Ann. § 1337.16 (B) (2)(b) (Anderson 2016); and Wyoming, Wyo. Stat. Ann. §35-22-408 (g) ii (Michie 2016).

Idaho requires life preserving treatment unless it would be futile. Oklahoma does not allow withholding treatment for the elderly, disabled, or terminally ill individual.
Idaho, Idaho Code § 39-4514 (2017), Oklahoma, 2016 Ok. ALS 160, 1 (2013), to be codified as 63 Okla. Stat. §§ 3090.3.

If not listed above, there are 21 states and territories that do not specify life preserving treatment be provided pending a patient's transfer. Where does that leave you or someone you love?

That is why it is so important when you are young and healthy to find out what the rules are that may impact your medical care and your life, and those you love.
It's all about Broken Trust in the health care system if you are in the "At Risk" or the Vulnerable Group.
If you don't protect yourself – they won't.

Don't let them decide how and when you die.

# Disclaimer

This booklet is presented for educational purposes only. Under no circumstances should it be mistaken for professional legal or medical advice, nor is it at all intended to be taken as such. The commentary and other contents simply reflect the opinion of the author alone. The presence of a link to a website does not indicate accuracy, approval or endorsement of that website or any services, products, or opinions that may be offered by them.

www.ingramcontent.com/pod-product-compliance
Lightning Source LLC
Chambersburg PA
CBHW050840290526
45792CB00001B/468